AF186664

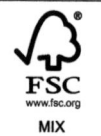

Microcirculation of Blood 101

The Next Generation of Healthcare

Peter Carl Simons

Bemer Products are made by Bemer International AG in Triesen

Bibliografische Information der Deutschen Nationalbibliothek:

Die Deutsche Nationalbibliothek verzeichnet diese Publikation in der Deutschen Nationalbibliografie; detaillierte bibliografische Daten sind im Internet über http://dnb.dnb.de abrufbar.

Herstellung und Verlag: BoD –
Books on Demand, Norderstedt

ISBN: 978-3-7519-5696-3

Introduction

By using this book, you accept this disclaimer in full.

No advice

The book contains information. The information is not advice and should not be treated as such.

No representations or warranties

To the maximum extent permitted by applicable law and subject to section below, we exclude all representations, warranties, undertakings and guarantees relating to the book.

Without prejudice to the generality of the foregoing paragraph, we do not represent, warrant, undertake or guarantee:

- that the information in the book is correct, accurate, complete or non-misleading.

- that the use of the guidance in the book will lead to any particular outcome or result.

Limitations and exclusions of liability

The limitations and exclusions of liability set out in this section and elsewhere in this disclaimer: are subject to section 6 below; and govern all liabilities arising under the disclaimer or in relation to the book, including liabilities arising in contract, in tort (including negligence) and for breach of statutory duty.

We will not be liable to you in respect of any losses arising out of any event or events beyond our reasonable control.

We will not be liable to you in respect of any business losses, including without limitation loss of or damage to profits, income, revenue, use, production, anticipated savings, business, contracts, commercial opportunities or goodwill.

We will not be liable to you in respect of any loss or corruption of any data, database or software.

We will not be liable to you in respect of any special, indirect or consequential loss or damage.

Exceptions

Nothing in this disclaimer shall: limit or exclude our liability for death or personal injury resulting from negligence; limit or exclude our liability for fraud or fraudulent misrepresentation; limit any of our liabilities in any way that is not permitted under applicable law; or exclude any of our liabilities that may not be excluded under applicable law.

Severability

If a section of this disclaimer is determined by any court or other competent authority to be unlawful and/or unenforceable, the other sections of this disclaimer continue in effect.

If any unlawful and/or unenforceable section would be lawful or enforceable if part of it were deleted, that part will be deemed to be deleted, and the rest of the section will continue in effect.

Law and jurisdiction

This disclaimer will be governed by and construed in accordance with Swiss law, and any disputes relating to this disclaimer will be subject to the exclusive jurisdiction of the courts of Switzerland.

Inhaltsverzeichnis

Inhaltsverzeichnis   **9**

What is Microcirculation?   **11**

The Main Sectors of Microcirculation   **14**

How Microcirculation is Regulated   **16**

Microcirculatory Exchange   *19*

How Capillary Exchange is Regulated   *21*

The Process of Diffusion in the Microcirculation of Blood
                                                            23

Bulk Flow   *25*

Transcytosis   *27*

The next generation of Healthcare   **29**

Hypertension and its Relation to Microcirculation   *30*

Normal Hydrostatic Pressure in the Bloodstream   *33*

Hydrostatic Pressure during Hypertension   *33*

*Hypertension and the Abnormalities in the
Microcirculatory System*   *34*

*How the Microcirculation System May Increase
Hypertension*   *36*

Using Microcirculation Knowledge in the Prevention of End-Organ Damage   *38*

Available Strategies in the Treatment of Hypertension at the Microcirculatory Level   *41*

Final Thoughts   **45**

Bemer Physical Vascular Therapy   **46**

Bemer Group Products   *47*

The BEMER Pro Set   *48*

The Classic Set   *50*

What is Microcirculation?

By definition, microcirculation of blood is the circulation of blood in the smallest of blood vessels which are present in the vasculature embedded in the organ tissues. The difference between microcirculation and macrocirculation is that the latter refers to the circulation of blood to and from body organs. For its part, the microcirculation of blood is made up of terminal venules, arterioles, and capillaries which work by draining capillary blood. The flow of blood at the microcirculation level flows from the arteries to the arterioles, through the capillaries and out through the venules and into the veins. The arterioles are innervated and surrounded all around by muscle cells that are smooth. The arterioles measure anything between 10-100 μm and they carry blood to the capillaries.

However, the capillaries are not surrounded by smooth muscle cells, are not innervated, and are smaller in diameter at 5-8 μm. The blood then flows from the capillaries to the venules. The venules have the largest diameter limit and measure between 10 to 200 μm. They have some smooth muscle cells around them but not as much as that found in the arterioles. From the venules, the blood flows to the veins. The three types of blood channels mentioned above are not the only ones involved in the microcirculation of blood. Other blood channels include collecting ducts and lymphatic capillaries. The purposes of microcirculation include delivering nutrients and oxygen to the blood tissues followed by the removal of carbon dioxide and other wastes from the tissues. This system also regulates tissue perfusion and blood flow and, in effect, has a direct influence on the blood pressure. Through the pericyte cells which have the capacity to contract and expand to vary the size of the arterioles thus the level of pressure for the blood flowing through the tissues. This same system also determines the responses to inflammation which may include swelling or edema.

The structure of the vessels involved in microcirculation has the flattened signature cells of the endothelium with many of them being surrounded by pericytes which are contractile cells. The nature of the endothelium allows it to act as a suitable surface for the smooth flow of blood. Its structure is also right for the regulation of the movement of dissolved minerals and water between the tissues and the blood in the interstitial plasma. The other purpose of the endothelium is the production of molecules that serve to prevent the clotting of blood. The molecules only cease working there is a leak, and clotting is deemed necessary to preserve the life of the individual.

The Main Sectors of Microcirculation

The microcirculation of blood has three main sectors namely the resistive (pre-capillary) sector, the swap (capillary) sector, and the capacitive (post-capillary) sector.

i. **Pre-capillary sector;** in this sector, there is participation from the pre-capillary sphincters and arterioles to regulate the flow of blood before it goes into the capillaries and venules. They work through relaxation and contraction mechanisms of the smooth muscles embedded in their walls.

ii. **Capillary sector;** probably the most important sector of the three mentioned above, the capillary sector involves the flow of blood through the capillaries. As the blood flows through the capillaries, gasses and substances are exchanged between the blood and the interstitial fluids in the tissues. Most importantly, oxygen and nutrients from the blood are absorbed into the interstitial fluids while carbon dioxide and wastes are moved into the blood. These exchanges occur across the walls of the capillaries.

iii. **Post-capillary sector;** the post-capillary sector is made up of the post-capillary venules that are formed from a layer of endothelial cells which also allow the movement of substances across them. From here, the blood flows to the veins and away from the organ in question.

How Microcirculation is Regulated

At the lowest level of blood circulation, there is a lot that goes on to regulate this process. The regulation of blood flow at this level also determines the flow of blood in the whole body. The process of tissue perfusion is carried out at the microcirculation level. At this level, the contraction and relaxation of the arterioles serve to control the blood flow through the capillaries. The contraction and relaxation of the arterioles vary the vascular tone and diameter of these blood vessels which translates to the various responses of the vascular smooth muscle to the various types of stimuli. If for example, the blood vessels become distended, there would be an increase in the level of pressure of the blood flowing to the tissues. This aspect serves as a stimulus for the arteriolar wall muscles to contract and regulate the pressure. If on the other hand, the blood vessels reduce in size and reduce the amount of blood pressure in the body, the arteriolar wall muscles will relax to allow in more blood into the tissues to a given constant. No matter what happens to the blood pressure of the body, the blood pressure in the tissues will be held at a constant through this process. All tissues in the body have this blood pressure regulation mechanism for uniformity of function given that the level of pressure in the body is the right one for the exchange of substances through the capillary walls with the tissues. Higher or lower blood temperature will hamper the effectiveness of this process.

The nervous system also regulates the microcirculation process. The sympathetic nervous system is vital in the activation of the smaller arterioles and terminals. The nervous system also plays the role of releasing   neurotransmitters, neuropeptides, and hormones such as adrenaline, noradrenaline, atrial natriuretic peptide, vasopressin, renin-angiotensin, and catecholamine which play vital roles in the regulation of the microcirculation process. All these hormones have varying effects on the microcirculation system as they cause vasoconstriction, vasodilation besides affecting the alpha and beta adrenergic receptors.

The working of the arterioles is actually simple yet fascinating as they occur at very microscopic levels. These arterioles work by responding to the metabolic stimuli secreted and generated in the specific tissues in the body. Vasodilation of the arterioles is triggered by the accumulation of catabolic products in the tissues. The catabolic products occur as a result of an increase in the level of metabolism in the tissues. Vasodilation enables the endothelium to control the tone of the muscle cells within it and the arteriolar blood flow tissue. The endothelium also has the task of circulating, activating and inactivating the contents of plasma such as the hormones. To vary the diameter of the vessels within the tissues to certain diameter levels, the endothelium secretes substances that act as the vasodilators and vasoconstrictors. Basically, the activities in the blood vessels in the tissues are the result of endothelium cells and their activities in response to the existing conditions in the body.

Microcirculatory Exchange

Also referred to as a capillary exchange, the microcirculatory exchange is the exchange of substances in the capillaries of the body. The capillaries are the smallest types of blood vessels besides being the highest in number too. Their high number is meant to ramify as much of the blood tissues as possible. It is also meant to reduce the distance required for the diffusion of substances into and out of the tissues of the body. Their thin walls make them the best in this process as they increase the surface area for the best exchange while reducing the time traveled by the substances being exchanged. The exchange between the blood and the interstitial fluid occurs in the 7% of the blood that is always in the capillaries at any time in the body. It is this exchange between the interstitial fluid and the blood that is named capillary exchange. The main processes by which the exchange occurs are vesicular transport (transcytosis), bulk flow, and diffusion. All the types of the tissues including the post-capillary venules, collecting venules, and the capillaries take place in the process of exchanging of the liquids and solids through the capillary walls. Besides the plasma proteins which are too big to pass through the capillary walls, everything else is exchanged through these walls. The kinetic motion of molecules is employed in the absorption of these unabsorbed proteins during the second passing through the capillaries (after the first pass has not absorbed them).

How Capillary Exchange is Regulated

There is an array of mechanisms which will go into the regulation of the microcirculatory mechanisms. Together, these mechanisms ensure that capillary exchange occurs as fast and as safely as possible.

i. **Diffusion;** the rate of diffusion rate, being inversely proportional to the distance between the capillaries and the cells, is reduced as much as possible. To achieve this, the capillaries are in large numbers such that each individual cell is close to a capillary vessel. To further reduce the diffusion distance, the capillaries have a small diameter such that the substances in the blood and the interstitial fluid have the shortest route possible.

ii. **Surface area;** the surface area for the diffusion is also immensely increased owing to the large number of capillaries in the body. The estimated number of the capillaries is at least 10 to 14 million. Even with that, at each time, only between 5 to 7% of the total amount of blood in the body is contained in the capillaries.

iii. **Blood pressure;** compared to other parts of the body, the blood in the capillaries is at its slowest. The slow pace is occasioned by the high amount of branching of the capillaries. The advantage with the relatively lower blood pressure is that it allows the exchange of substances to take place effectively and at a faster rate than if the blood was flowing faster.

The Process of Diffusion in the Microcirculation of Blood

Of the three processes that enable the exchange of materials between the blood and the interstitial fluid, diffusion is responsible for the largest part of the exchange process. Diffusion is a process by which molecules move to regions where they are less concentrated from regions where they have a higher concentration level. For diffusion to work, therefore, there have to be differences between the concentration of the substances in the blood and the interstitial fluid. When compared to the interstitial fluids, the blood has a higher concentration of the substances needed by the cells such as oxygen, amino acids, glucose and others. These substances will thus move from the blood to the interstitial fluid. On the contrary, the interstitial fluid is richer in wastes such as carbon dioxide compared to the blood. The wastes would thus diffuse from the interstitial fluid into the bloodstream inside the capillaries. The formation of the endothelium will determine the extent to which the capillary walls are permeable. The arrangement of the endothelial cells can be fenestrated, continuous or discontinuous with their level of permeability. This level of permeability is what determines the substances that will pass across the endothelial cells and which ones will not. Other forces which play a role in the exchange process and are related to diffusion are osmosis and hydrostatic force. Together, these forces are referred as the Starling forces and their role is well documented using the Starling equation.

Bulk Flow

Bulk flow is the movement of substances across the capillary walls in bulk rather than in small dissolved amounts. For the substances which are not soluble in lipids, bulk flow is the only way they can move across the capillary walls. Again, the permeability of the capillary walls determines the level of bulk flow. The permeability also relies on the structure of the cells in the capillary walls. For example, when the capillaries have a tight structure to form a continuous capillary wall, the level of bulk flow will be significantly reduced. However, when the capillary walls are perforated owing to having a fenestrated cell structure, the level of bulk flow will be significantly increased. The best capillary cell structure is the discontinuous capillaries which have great intercellular gaps for ease of passage of the substances that will not dissolve in lipids. The pressure differences between the bloodstream and the interstitial space (interstitium) play a major role in the process of bulk flow. For instance, when the substances move from the blood to the interstitial space, it will be due to the blood hydrostatic pressure (BHP) and the interstitial fluid osmotic pressure (IFOP). This process is referred to as filtration. The inverse of filtration is referred to as reabsorption, and it involves the movement of substances by bulk flow from the interstitial space into the bloodstream. Reabsorption is a result of the differences in pressure caused by the blood colloid pressure (BCOP) and the interstitial fluid hydrostatic pressure (IFHP). The determinant of whether a substance will be reabsorbed or filtered is the differences in the four types of pressures. This difference is known as the net filtration pressure (NFP). To obtain the net filtration pressure, one has to balance out the hydrostatic pressures (BHP and IFHP) and the osmotic pressures (IFOP and BCOP). The four types of pressures make what is called the Starling forces. If the value of the net filtration pressure is positive, the process that will occur will be filtration. On the other hand, if the result of the net filtration pressure is negative, the process to expect is that if reabsorption.

Transcytosis

The third and last mechanism of capillary exchange is that of transcytosis. Also called vesicular transport, transcytosis involves the movement of large substances across the endothelial cells of the capillary walls. First of all, the substances move into the interstitial space from the bloodstream. When the substances exit the interstitial space, they do so through the process of exocytosis. This process is well suited to the substances which are not soluble in lipids among them hormones such as insulin. The movement of substances from the cell into the interstitial space using the process of transcytosis requires vesicles to and from the capillaries. Once the vesicles leave the cells, they may either merge to mix their contents or go to specific tissues directly. Intermixed materials increase the functional capability of the vesicles.

The next generation of Healthcare

Nowadays, there is a lot going on in the field of medicine. One of the most common problems realized is that of hypertension. More and more people are reporting the failure of their bodies in controlling the pressure of the blood in their bodies. When the body has too much pressure in its vessels, there will be a problem in the control of most body processes. Although previous methods in controlling the pressure of the body focused on controlling the activity of the heart and other internal organs, the next generation of healthcare will focus on the microcirculation process to control the pressure of the body. The role of the microcirculation process in the control of hypertension is the new focus for most scientists who have realized that this small scale process determines the general pressure of the body to a large extent.

Hypertension and its Relation to Microcirculation

Hypertension adversely affects the process of microcirculation. There are three major ways by which this health condition will render the process of microcirculation ineffective.

i.   Hypertension may render the processes controlling the vasomotor tone abnormal such that their levels of responses are hampered. In this way, they may have too much vasoconstriction or too little vasodilation. The blood pressure within them will thus be mostly abnormal in response to the blood pressure of the rest of the body.

ii.   Hypertension can also affect the
        structure of the microcirculatory
        vessels, for example, through in-
        crease the ratio of the wall to the
        lumen of these vessels. The
        change in structure will be
        accompanied by changes in the
        pressure of the blood flowing
        within them.

iii.   Hypertension is also likely to cause
        changes in the microvascular net-
        works such as the increase or re-
        duction (rarefaction) in the den-
        sity of the capillaries and arteri-
        oles. This change will have a
        significant change on the level of
        blood pressure in the microcircula-
        tory vessels.

The three ways hypertension affects the microcirculation system can be directly related

to the path followed by antihypertensive therapists and their methodologies in alleviating this conditions. First of all, antihypertensive therapy was focused on the alteration of the vasomotor tone and the promotion of vasodilation. As the times went by, the focus shifted more on the reduction of the resistance created by the vessel structures. Lastly and most recently, the focus has been on the correction of the changes brought about by the changes in the density of the microvascular network. The problem has been that some antihypertensive agents working to reduce the vasomotor tone have chronic actions on the vessels in the body and thus hampering their effectiveness in helping manage hypertension.

Normal Hydrostatic Pressure in the Bloodstream

There are lower and higher limits of the blood pressure of the blood in the various vessels in the body. It drops when entering the microcirculation system and rises again when leaving it. The entry and exit pressure values of the blood into and out of the vessels are approximately the same.

Hydrostatic Pressure during Hypertension

During hypertension, there are various changes that occur in the body. First, when the blood is leaving the heart, the pressure remains the same as during normal blood pressure conditions. However, there is a distinguished increase in the peripheral vascular resistance to the flow of blood leading to the increase in the pressure level of the body. In the precapillary vasculature, the pressure of blood is proportionally increased. Also, there is a noted drop in the blood pressure in the arterioles and the arteries with these vessels also experiencing increased resistance during hypertension.

Hypertension and the Abnormalities in the Microcirculatory System

The small arteries in the body vary their diameter in accordance with the external blood pressure in order to keep the blood pressure in the tissues at a constant level. However, during hypertension, the diameters of these arteries have been noted to decrease significantly. Also noted severally is the increase in the media to lumen ratio for the small arteries. Both cases are not safe for the human body as they affect the pressure of the blood flowing in the tissues.

The most dangerous cases noted focused on the discovery that, during hypertension, there is a significant reduction in the density or number of microvessels. The reduction in the density and the number of microvessels takes various stages with the first one involving their constriction owing to their sensitivity to the vasoconstriction stimuli having been heightened. This constriction is so extreme that they become unable to allow nonperfusion. The second stage involves further constriction to the extent that they eventually disappear. This case can be seen in patients with primary hypertension who experience a reduction in the capillaries in their fingers. One needs to be watchful when making a diagnosis of hypertension since the same process can be experienced when the individual has hypertrophic cardiomyopathy, syndrome X, or scleroderma. Only when other symptoms of hypertension have been confirmed will the individual be termed to be hypertensive. The problem brought about by the reduction in the number and density of the blood vessels is that there is a notable reduction in the surface area for the exchange of substances between the blood and the interstitial fluid. Also, microvascular rarefaction increases the distance between the cells and vessels thus making the processes of exchanging the substances difficult and significantly slow.

How the Microcirculation System May Increase Hypertension

The microvascular system has various contributions to the existence and prevalence of hypertension. As a matter of fact, hypertension and the microvascular system may work hand in hand in increasing the blood pressure in the body. The microcirculation system responds to increases in the blood pressure by constricting in order to keep the blood pressure in the tissues at a constant level. The problem is that this same constricting mechanism serves to increase the blood pressure in the body. A vicious cycle thus ensues leading a long-term increase in the blood pressure of the whole body from a small increase. A study on this issue led scientists to conclude that there is concrete evidence between the birth weight and the placental weight of the people in the study group. Those born as small babies but with large placentas recorded the highest level of blood pressure. The explanations given were that the reduced flow of blood in the trunk of a fetus which is small in size in relation to the placenta might lead to the reduction in the growth of the microcirculatory system. Such babies are likely to have hypertension when they are adults. The second explanation for the same findings was that, when the development of the microcirculatory system is impaired, the chances of the baby developing anomalies are significantly increased. The anomalies may, later on, manifest themselves as increased blood pressure.

Using Microcirculation Knowledge in the Prevention of End-Organ Damage

When administered well, most forms of anti-hypertensive therapy have proven effective in the reduction and prevention of certain circulatory problems such as coronary heart disease and stroke. The problem has been that most of the conditions causing end-organ damage such as microvascular angina, lacunar infarction, retinopathy, and nephropathy involve hypertension and the microcirculation system. Therefore, in efforts geared towards preventing hypertension and other issues, the individual can benefit from the prevention of end-organ damage.

1. **Microalbuminuria;** microalbuminuria, also referred to as increased albumin excretion, is one of the major risk factors for cardiovascular disease and death both in individuals with or without diabetes. A study established the fact that there was a higher chance of having proteinuria in patients with hypertension than those without. The results pointed to 3 times the chance of hypertensive patients having proteinuria compared to normotensive ones. The same results translate to hypertensive patients with proteinuria being three times more likely to than normal ones. The good news is that microalbuminuria is a reversible condition.

2. **Microcirculation in the Myocardium;** although the structure of the heart is among the most reliable in terms of preventing end-organ damage, the heart may still suffer from end-organ

damage especially when there are changes in the microvessel structure in the heart. When the myocardial microvascular structure does not develop well in the fetus, and as it grows up, there is the increased risk of end-organ damage in the heart.

3. **Cerebral Microcirculation;** when one is a patient of hypertension, they are predisposed to a very high chance of stroke. The occurrence of deep but tiny infarcts from the rupture of small veins or occlusion in what is called lacunar infarction is the cause of stroke in most patients with hypertension. Hypertension causes various changes in the cerebral arteriolar structure as evidenced by the increase in the media to lumen ratio and the reduction in the diameter of the vessels. The good news is that studies have proven the fact that hypertension does not cause the rarefaction of

capillaries or cerebral arterioles. The better news is that some types of antihypertensive therapy has been proven to reverse the negative changes in the structure of the cerebral microvessel thus reducing the chances of stroke.

Available Strategies in the Treatment of Hypertension at the Microcirculatory Level

When targeting the microcirculation structure in treating hypertension and preventing end-organ damage, the focus is on reducing the wall to lumen ratio and reversing the microvascular rarefaction. Among the most common antihypertensive agents are outlined here;

1. **Diurectics;** the use of hydrochlorothiazide therapy has proven to be very

ineffective in the restoration of the structure of the microvessels.

2. **Beta-Blockers (β-Blockers);** beta-blockers have proven to have but little effect in restoring the structural changes in the microvessels of the body. Among the most common beta-blockers are atenolol and propranolol which have shown little success in treating the effects of hypertension on the microcirculatory system.

3. **Alpha-Blockers (α-Blockers);** alpha-blockers have shown promising results in experimental setups, α-adrenoreceptor blockade agents like prazosin has proved to lead to the increased density I the density of the capillaries in the body.

4. **Calcium Antagonists;** calcium antagonists have proven to be very effective in the restoration of the structure of the microvessels with variants such as verapamil, nifedipine and nimodipine

all showing excellent results in this test.

5. **ACE Inhibitors;** although mixed, the results in using ACE inhibitors have been generally positive in the inhibition of ACE activity. Thus ACE inhibitors can play a vital role in the reduction of the media to lumen ratio in the microvessels. However, the same ACE inhibitors have been found to reduce the density of the venules and arterioles in the body tissues which is not a positive sign of their effectiveness. The results for the uses of ACE inhibitors, therefore, are mixed in many ways and need further research before they can be put to good use.

6. **Combination therapy;** the use of various methods to counteract the effects of hypertension and the end-organ damage have been immensely effective. For example the combination of beta-blockers and ACE inhibitors

than when either therapy was used on its own. Also, combining an ACE inhibitor called perindopril with diuretic indapamide has proven to increase the diameter and capillary density of the microvessels.

Final Thoughts

The microcirculation system plays a very important role in the body. Through this process, the body tissues get nutrients and oxygen delivered to them for proper functioning. Also, the same system ensures that the wastes created by the functioning of the cells are taken away to reduce the chances of the death of the cells from the accumulation of wastes. The microcirculation system keeps the pressure of blood in the tissues and organs at a consistent level through the processes of vasodilation and vasoconstriction of these vessels. However, during bodily anomalies such as hypertension, the function of this system is greatly hampered with the solution to restoring normal functioning being possible only through the use of antihypertensive agents.

Bemer Physical Vascular Therapy

The Bemer Group offers among the best equipment to alleviate microcirculation issues. The firm has been in operation for quite some time as evidenced by its various documentations among them an ISO 13485 certification and a reddot design award (2013). The company has made a name for itself as the leading provider of physical vascular therapy which geared towards supporting the body to heal itself in terms of restoring the natural structure of the vessels involved in the microcirculation system.

With the Bemer Group, one will be in the hands of highly qualified medical personnel to deal with the health problems they have. For the most part, the methods employed by this group have been protected by patents owing to the amount of research that has gone into them. As time goes by, the company's researchers also incorporate the latest findings in the field of microcirculation into the equipment and methods used. This aspect ensures that the patients get the best healthcare from the Bemer Group.

Bemer Group Products

The Bemer Group offers two main types of products namely The BEMER Pro Set and The Classic Set. Besides that, there is an array of application modules such as the comfort chair (B.COMFORT), Light Treatment (B.LIGHT), Small-Scale treatment (B.PAD), Selective treatment (B.SPOT), Seat cushion (B.SIT), Full Body treatment (B.BODY Pro), and the Full Body treatment (B.BODY Classic). All these application modules come together with the various accessories to ensure that the machines mentioned above work accordingly for the best results. The accessories include Handle (B.GRIP), Fixing strap, Wall mounting, foot protection, protection glasses, power supply unit, car power cable, signal tester (B.SCAN), and the rechargeable battery that powers the machines in the case that the power grid is not behaving accordingly.

The BEMER Pro Set

This is the ultimate all-in-one solution for Physical Vascular Therapy. It has all the tools and capabilities one would need when dealing with their physical vascular therapy. The Bemer Group's reddot design award clearly comes out in this machine for its great ergonomics and sleek design. The touch screen has easy to use items which are clearly arranged that one can easily see the options they need to select to effect the treatment. With the touch of a finger, one can start their treatment for the best results when using this machine. There are no complex commands or signals on the touchscreen display. The commands on the display will guide the individual through the treatment steps which can be performed with lots of ease. The good news is that the large display can be used to control two machines at the same time when using the 2-in-1 function that comes bundled with it. No need to obtain two control panels when with the included control. It also features a wide range of accessories and application modules to enhance its use in the provision of physical vascular therapy. The BEMER Pro Set works by harnessing the application modules in the conducting of the BEMER signal which is generated in the control unit. The control unit is allows for the treatment of the exact areas of the body which are in need of the treatment.

Besides the normal standardized treatment programs which can be applied as needed, the BEMER Pro Set also comes bundled with

3 pre-set programs which work by facilitating the intensive treatment of specific areas. The areas to be treated can be selected from the B.BOX control unit with 10 intensity levels to choose from. The BEMER Pro Set has many other functions and capabilities.

The Classic Set

The Classic Set from the Bemer Group is aimed at those who are starting out on the physical vascular treatment program. It has many benefits including an easy to use interface on the graphic display, a three-step program for versatility of use, ten different levels of treatment intensity, and a sleep and regeneration program meant to allow the body recover from the treatment. The whole set can be obtained from the company's online platform.